Celiac Disease

An Autoimmune Disorder Triggered by Gluten

Comprehensive Guide to Managing Celiac Disease, Gluten Sensitivity, and Living a Gluten-Free Lifestyle for Long-Term Health

Graham Julian Oliver

Disclaimer

The information provided in this book, *Celiac Disease – An Autoimmune Disorder Triggered by Gluten*, is intended for educational and informational purposes only. It is not a substitute for professional medical advice, diagnosis, or treatment. Always seek the advice of your physician or other qualified health provider with any questions you may have regarding a medical condition or treatment.

The author and publisher of this book make no representations or warranties with respect to the accuracy, applicability, fitness, or completeness of the contents. Any reliance you place on such information is strictly at your own risk.

Additionally, the author does not endorse any specific individual, product, website, organization, or other names that may be referenced or mentioned in this book. Any references made are solely for informational purposes and should not be construed as endorsements.

About This Book

The book "Celiac Disease – An Autoimmune Disorder Triggered by Gluten: Comprehensive Guide to Managing Celiac Disease, Gluten Sensitivity, and Living a Gluten-Free Lifestyle for Long-Term Health" serves as an essential resource for anyone grappling with the complexities of celiac disease and gluten sensitivity. This comprehensive guide is not merely a compilation of facts but an empowering tool designed to enhance understanding and promote effective management of celiac disease. It meticulously details the nature of the disorder, explaining how gluten acts as a trigger for symptoms and damage in the small intestine, emphasizing the importance of a strict gluten-free diet as a cornerstone for symptom management and healing.

This book goes beyond mere definitions and symptoms; it dives into the nuanced differences between celiac disease and gluten sensitivity while also addressing genetic and environmental factors contributing to the condition. It provides clarity on diagnosis methods, including blood tests and biopsies, underscoring the detrimental effects of undiagnosed celiac disease on overall health. Addressing common misconceptions, the book highlights the importance of early diagnosis and treatment and explores the complex relationship between celiac disease and other autoimmune disorders. Readers will gain insight into the long-term complications of untreated celiac disease and the vital role healthcare providers play in managing this condition. It encourages readers to seek out support groups and resources, fostering a sense of community that is often crucial for those navigating this journey.

As the guide progresses, it seamlessly transitions into practical aspects of living gluten-free, detailing essential steps for adopting a gluten-free diet. It offers thorough instructions on identifying gluten-containing grains, understanding gluten-free alternatives, and the importance of reading food labels for hidden gluten. Moreover, it emphasizes the risks of cross-contamination and provides invaluable cooking methods to ensure a safe gluten-free kitchen. The book serves as a treasure trove of meal planning strategies and shopping tips that empower readers to create a dedicated gluten-free pantry, simplifying the transition to a gluten-free lifestyle.

Nutritional considerations are another focal point, with the book illuminating key nutrients often lacking in a gluten-free diet and stressing the importance of whole foods over processed alternatives. It encourages incorporating a variety of fruits, vegetables, and protein sources while also highlighting essential vitamins and minerals for individuals with celiac disease. The text recognizes that maintaining hydration and balancing electrolytes are critical, and it provides strategies for achieving a nutritionally balanced diet, including the importance of consulting with a dietitian.

The guide also offers a wealth of information on cooking and baking gluten-free, providing essential techniques and tips for using gluten-free flours effectively. It addresses common mistakes in gluten-free baking and encourages creativity in meal prep, ensuring that readers can enjoy delicious, safe meals without compromising on taste.

Understanding the challenges of dining out and navigating social situations is paramount, and this book equips readers with strategies for effectively communicating dietary needs in restaurants, finding gluten-free eateries, and preparing for social events. It addresses the emotional aspects of living with celiac disease, including anxiety around food and the importance of building a supportive network. By providing practical strategies for coping with frustration and isolation, the book fosters resilience and encourages a positive relationship with food.

In an ever-evolving field, the importance of staying informed cannot be overstated. This guide emphasizes the value of ongoing education about celiac disease, keeping readers updated on the latest research and developments, and engaging with advocacy organizations and gluten-free communities. It encourages sharing personal experiences to foster awareness and understanding within one's social circles, thus contributing to a broader cultural shift towards greater acceptance of gluten-free lifestyles.

Overall, this comprehensive guide not only aims to educate and inform but also inspires confidence in those living with celiac disease and gluten sensitivity. By equipping readers with knowledge and practical strategies, it empowers them to embrace a gluten-free lifestyle, manage their health effectively, and thrive in their personal and social lives.

Table of Contents

Celiac Disease – An Autoimmune Disorder Triggered by Gluten

Definition and Overview of Celiac Disease

Celiac disease is a chronic autoimmune disorder that occurs in genetically predisposed individuals. When gluten, a protein found in wheat, barley, and rye, is ingested, the immune system mistakenly attacks the lining of the small intestine, leading to inflammation and damage. This can result in a range of symptoms, including digestive issues, fatigue, and nutrient deficiencies. It's crucial for those experiencing symptoms related to gluten consumption to seek medical advice for proper testing and diagnosis.

Understanding celiac disease is vital for managing it effectively. Once diagnosed, individuals must adopt a gluten-free lifestyle to prevent symptoms and long-term health complications. This guide will help readers navigate the complexities of living with celiac disease, providing them with the knowledge and tools needed for a successful gluten-free journey.

The Role of Gluten in Triggering Symptoms and Damage in the Small Intestine

Gluten is a mixture of proteins found in certain grains that can trigger adverse reactions in individuals with celiac disease. When consumed, gluten can provoke an immune response that damages the villi, small finger-like projections lining the intestine, which are essential for nutrient absorption. This damage can lead to various gastrointestinal symptoms, including bloating, diarrhea, and abdominal pain, as well as non-gastrointestinal symptoms such as skin rashes and neurological issues.

To mitigate these effects, it's crucial to understand how gluten interacts with the body. Identifying gluten-containing foods and understanding their impact on the immune system helps individuals with celiac disease make informed dietary choices. This awareness will empower readers to recognize the importance of avoiding gluten to promote healing and overall health.

Importance of a Strict Gluten-Free Diet for Symptom Management and Healing

A strict gluten-free diet is the cornerstone of managing celiac disease. By completely eliminating gluten from the diet, individuals can significantly reduce inflammation in the intestines, allowing the damaged tissue to heal and alleviating symptoms. This process may involve reading food labels carefully, avoiding cross-contamination, and seeking gluten-free alternatives to favorite foods, ensuring that every meal is safe and nourishing.

To maintain a successful gluten-free diet, meal planning and preparation are essential. Readers should familiarize themselves with gluten-free grains like quinoa, rice, and corn, and focus on whole, unprocessed foods, such as fruits, vegetables, lean meats, and legumes. Developing these habits will support long-term health and well-being while preventing accidental gluten exposure.

Overview of the Book's Structure and How to Use It for Effective Management of Celiac Disease

This book is structured to provide a comprehensive resource for individuals managing celiac disease and gluten sensitivity. Each chapter covers critical aspects, including dietary recommendations, meal planning, and coping strategies, making it easy to navigate and find relevant information. Readers can use the table of contents to quickly locate topics of interest, enabling them to focus on their unique needs and circumstances.

To get the most out of this guide, readers should approach it as both an educational tool and a practical reference. By engaging with each chapter, they can build a strong foundation for understanding celiac disease, learn to avoid gluten effectively, and develop strategies for living a fulfilling gluten-free life.

CHAPTER 1:

Understanding Celiac Disease

Symptoms and Signs of Celiac Disease

Celiac disease manifests through various symptoms, including gastrointestinal issues like diarrhea, bloating, and abdominal pain. Other signs can include fatigue, unexplained weight loss, and skin rashes. Some individuals may experience neurological symptoms, such as headaches or mood disorders, making it vital to recognize that symptoms can vary widely between individuals.

To identify potential celiac disease, keep a detailed symptom diary, noting when symptoms occur and any foods consumed. This record can help healthcare providers better understand your condition and recommend appropriate testing if celiac disease is suspected.

Difference between Celiac Disease and Gluten Sensitivity

Celiac disease is an autoimmune disorder triggered by gluten, leading to intestinal damage and other health issues. In contrast, gluten sensitivity may cause similar gastrointestinal symptoms without the autoimmune response or damage to the intestines. Understanding this distinction is crucial for appropriate dietary management and treatment.

If you suspect gluten sensitivity, consult a healthcare professional for guidance. They may recommend eliminating gluten from your diet temporarily to observe symptom improvement, while celiac disease requires strict, lifelong avoidance of gluten.

Genetic and Environmental Factors Contributing to Celiac Disease

Celiac disease has a genetic component, meaning it often runs in families. Specific genes, such as HLA-DQ2 and HLA-DQ8, increase the risk of developing the condition. Environmental factors, including gastrointestinal infections, diet during infancy, and changes in gut bacteria, can also trigger the onset of celiac disease in genetically predisposed individuals.

To assess your risk, discuss your family history with your healthcare provider. They can suggest genetic testing if you have a family member with celiac disease, helping you understand your potential susceptibility and take preventative measures.

Diagnosis Methods: Blood Tests and Biopsy

Diagnosing celiac disease typically begins with blood tests to measure specific antibodies associated with the disorder, such as tissue transglutaminase (tTG) antibodies. If these tests indicate celiac disease, a biopsy of the small intestine is usually performed to confirm intestinal damage.

To ensure accurate results, continue consuming gluten before testing. Avoiding gluten prematurely can lead to false negatives, delaying diagnosis and necessary treatment. Follow your healthcare provider's instructions for the testing process.

The Impact of Undiagnosed Celiac Disease on Health

Living with undiagnosed celiac disease can lead to severe health issues, including malnutrition, osteoporosis, and increased risk of certain cancers. The body's inability to absorb nutrients due to intestinal damage can cause a range of symptoms affecting overall well-being.

If you suspect celiac disease, seek medical evaluation promptly. Early diagnosis can help prevent complications and improve quality of life by allowing you to adopt a gluten-free diet and restore intestinal health.

Common Misconceptions About Celiac Disease

Many misconceptions surround celiac disease, such as the belief that it is just a food allergy or that it can be outgrown. Unlike food allergies, celiac disease is a lifelong condition requiring strict avoidance of gluten to prevent damage to the intestines and related health issues.

Educating yourself and others about celiac disease is essential. Reliable sources, including healthcare providers and reputable organizations, can provide accurate information to help dispel myths and promote understanding of the disorder.

The Importance of Early Diagnosis and Treatment

Early diagnosis and treatment of celiac disease are crucial to prevent long-term health complications. A strict gluten-free diet can significantly improve symptoms, promote healing of the intestine, and reduce the risk of associated health issues.

If you experience symptoms consistent with celiac disease, consult a healthcare professional promptly. Early intervention not only improves health outcomes but also enhances overall quality of life by reducing the burden of symptoms and complications.

How Celiac Disease Affects Children vs. Adults

Celiac disease can affect individuals of all ages, but symptoms may present differently in children compared to adults. In children, symptoms often include growth delays, irritability, and behavioral changes. Adults may experience more varied symptoms, including fatigue and skin issues, often leading to misdiagnosis.

If a child is diagnosed with celiac disease, it's essential to educate both the child and family about maintaining a gluten-free diet. For adults, understanding the diverse symptoms can help facilitate proper diagnosis and management.

The Relationship Between Celiac Disease and Other Autoimmune Disorders

Individuals with celiac disease have a higher likelihood of developing other autoimmune disorders, such as Type 1 diabetes and autoimmune thyroid disease. The shared genetic and environmental factors contribute to this increased risk, making awareness important for effective management.

If you have celiac disease, monitor for symptoms of other autoimmune conditions. Regular check-ups with healthcare providers can help detect and manage additional disorders early on, improving overall health outcomes.

Long-Term Complications of Untreated Celiac Disease

Untreated celiac disease can lead to several long-term complications, including severe nutritional deficiencies, osteoporosis, and an increased risk of intestinal lymphoma. These complications arise due to chronic inflammation and damage to the intestines, underscoring the importance of strict adherence to a gluten-free diet.

To mitigate these risks, regular follow-ups with a healthcare provider are essential. They can monitor your health, evaluate any complications, and adjust your diet or supplements as necessary to ensure optimal nutrition and health outcomes.

Role of Healthcare Providers in Managing Celiac Disease

Healthcare providers play a crucial role in diagnosing and managing celiac disease, providing guidance on a gluten-free diet, and monitoring overall health. They can offer personalized treatment plans, dietary advice, and referrals to specialists if needed.

To ensure effective management, maintain open communication with your healthcare provider. Regular check-ups and discussions about symptoms, dietary challenges, and health changes are vital for long-term success in managing celiac disease.

Importance of Support Groups and Resources

Support groups and resources are invaluable for individuals with celiac disease, offering community, shared experiences, and practical advice for navigating a gluten-free lifestyle. Connecting with others who understand the challenges can provide emotional support and enhance coping strategies.

Seek out local or online support groups focused on celiac disease. Educational resources, cooking classes, and forums can help empower you to live well with celiac disease, providing tools and tips to thrive in a gluten-free environment.

CHAPTER 2:

Adopting a Gluten-Free Diet

Understanding What Gluten Is and Where It's Found

Gluten is a protein found primarily in wheat, barley, and rye. It helps foods maintain their shape, acting as a glue that holds them together. Common sources of gluten include bread, pasta, cereals, and many processed foods. Additionally, gluten can be found in unexpected places, such as sauces, dressings, and even some medications, making it crucial for individuals with celiac disease to be vigilant.

To identify gluten in your diet, start by familiarizing yourself with the foods that typically contain it. Read ingredient lists carefully, and be aware that terms like "wheat flour," "barley malt," and "rye" indicate the presence of gluten. Knowing where gluten lurks will help you avoid accidental ingestion and support your transition to a gluten-free lifestyle.

Essential Steps for Going Gluten-Free

The first step in going gluten-free is to eliminate all sources of gluten from your diet. Begin by cleaning out your pantry and refrigerator of gluten-containing products, replacing them with gluten-free options. This includes grains, baked goods, and snacks. It's essential to educate yourself about gluten-free alternatives that provide similar textures and flavors.

Next, develop a meal plan that emphasizes whole, unprocessed foods like fruits, vegetables, lean proteins, and gluten-free grains such as quinoa or rice. Preparing your meals at home gives you better control over what you're consuming. Meal prepping can simplify this process, making it easier to stick to your new diet.

Identifying Gluten-Containing Grains

Recognizing which grains contain gluten is vital for anyone with celiac disease. The primary gluten-containing grains include wheat (in all forms), barley, and rye. This encompasses a wide range of products, from bread and pasta to beer and certain sauces. Understanding these sources will help you make informed food choices.

To further identify gluten-containing grains, learn about their different varieties. For instance, spelt and durum wheat are also forms of wheat and should be avoided. When shopping or dining out, ask questions about ingredients to ensure that you're steering clear of gluten in your meals.

Overview of Gluten-Free Grains and Substitutes

There are several grains and starches that are naturally gluten-free, including rice, corn, quinoa, and millet. These alternatives provide essential nutrients and can be used in a variety of recipes. For example, quinoa can serve as a protein-rich base for salads, while rice can replace pasta in many dishes.

In addition to whole grains, many gluten-free substitutes are available for baking and cooking. Almond flour, coconut flour, and gluten-free all-purpose flour blends can help you create baked goods that are just as delicious as their gluten-containing counterparts. Experimenting with these substitutes can broaden your gluten-free cooking repertoire.

Reading Food Labels for Hidden Gluten

When shopping for gluten-free foods, reading labels is crucial. The U.S. Food and Drug Administration (FDA) mandates that products labeled "gluten-free" must contain less than 20 parts per million of gluten. Look for this label to ensure you are choosing safe products. Additionally, be cautious of items that may contain gluten, as gluten can be present in sauces, dressings, and processed foods.

Pay attention to ingredient lists for hidden sources of gluten. Ingredients like malt, modified food starch, and flavorings can often contain gluten, so it's essential to be knowledgeable about these terms. If you're unsure about a product, contact the manufacturer for clarification.

Cross-Contamination: Risks and Prevention

Cross-contamination is a significant risk for individuals with celiac disease. This occurs when gluten-free foods come into contact with gluten-containing foods, either during cooking or serving. To prevent this, use separate utensils, cutting boards, and cooking surfaces for gluten-free food preparation.

Additionally, be cautious in shared spaces like restaurants or communal kitchens. Always communicate your dietary restrictions to restaurant staff and inquire about their gluten-free practices. By being proactive about cross-contamination, you can significantly reduce the risk of gluten exposure.

Cooking Methods to Avoid Gluten Contamination

Adopting safe cooking practices is essential for maintaining a gluten-free kitchen. Use dedicated pots, pans, and utensils for gluten-free cooking to prevent any contamination. If you share kitchen space with others who consume gluten, make sure to wash these items thoroughly before and after use.

When cooking, consider methods that inherently avoid gluten contamination, such as grilling, steaming, or baking. Always be mindful of the preparation surfaces you use, as flour from gluten-containing foods can linger and contaminate gluten-free ingredients.

Meal Planning for a Gluten-Free Lifestyle

Effective meal planning is key to successfully navigating a gluten-free lifestyle. Start by creating a weekly menu that includes a variety of gluten-free foods, ensuring a balanced diet rich in nutrients. Incorporate a mix of proteins, vegetables, and gluten-free grains to keep meals interesting and satisfying.

Utilize batch cooking to save time during the week. Prepare larger portions of gluten-free meals and store them in portioned containers for quick access. This strategy not only helps maintain a gluten-free diet but also minimizes the temptation to revert to gluten-containing convenience foods.

Shopping Tips for Gluten-Free Foods

When shopping for gluten-free products, familiarize yourself with brands that specialize in gluten-free foods. Many stores now have dedicated gluten-free aisles or sections, making it easier to find safe options. Always review labels carefully and opt for products with gluten-free certifications to ensure safety.

Consider shopping at health food stores or farmers' markets, where fresh, whole foods are available. Incorporating fruits, vegetables, and gluten-free grains into your diet can help you avoid processed foods that may contain hidden gluten. Be proactive in seeking out new products and experimenting with different brands to find what you enjoy.

Gluten-Free Alternatives for Common Ingredients

Finding gluten-free alternatives for common cooking and baking ingredients is essential for maintaining a gluten-free diet. For instance, instead of traditional wheat flour, you can use almond flour, coconut flour, or gluten-free flour blends. These alternatives can be utilized in various recipes, from pancakes to cookies.

In addition to flour substitutes, there are gluten-free options for breadcrumbs, pasta, and sauces. For instance, gluten-free breadcrumbs can be made from crushed gluten-free crackers or bread, while zucchini or spaghetti squash can serve as a pasta alternative. Experimenting with these substitutes will help you maintain familiar flavors and textures in your meals.

Importance of Dedicated Gluten-Free Kitchen Tools

Utilizing dedicated gluten-free kitchen tools is crucial for preventing cross-contamination. Consider investing in separate cutting boards, utensils, and storage containers for gluten-free food preparation. Labeling these items can further ensure they are used exclusively for gluten-free cooking.

Additionally, consider using gluten-free baking pans and cookware. Silicone bakeware and glass containers are great options as they are less likely to retain gluten residues compared to traditional metal pans. Having dedicated tools creates a safe environment for preparing gluten-free meals and fosters confidence in your cooking.

Understanding Gluten-Free Certifications on Products

Gluten-free certifications help consumers identify safe products. Look for labels that indicate a product has been tested and certified by recognized organizations, such as the Gluten-Free Certification Organization (GFCO) or the Celiac Support Association (CSA). These certifications typically ensure that the product meets strict gluten-free standards.

Familiarizing yourself with these certifications will make shopping easier and safer. When in doubt, check the manufacturer's website or contact them directly for information on their gluten-free practices. Understanding these certifications empowers you to make informed choices that support your health.

Building a Gluten-Free Pantry

Building a gluten-free pantry involves stocking up on safe, versatile ingredients that will support your cooking needs. Begin by including essential gluten-free grains, such as rice, quinoa, and oats. Additionally, incorporate gluten-free flours, canned beans, and legumes to create hearty meals.

Organize your pantry by keeping gluten-free items separate from gluten-containing foods. Label containers clearly and consider creating a shopping list of gluten-free staples to simplify your grocery trips. By maintaining a well-stocked gluten-free pantry, you'll always have the ingredients necessary to prepare delicious and safe meals.

CHAPTER 3:

Nutritional Considerations for Celiac Disease

Key Nutrients That May Be Lacking in a Gluten-Free Diet

A gluten-free diet can sometimes lead to deficiencies in essential nutrients typically found in whole grains, such as B vitamins, iron, calcium, and magnesium. To counteract this, it's crucial to include naturally gluten-free whole foods like quinoa, brown rice, and millet, which can help provide these missing nutrients. Additionally, consider fortified gluten-free products that may contain added vitamins and minerals.

To ensure you're getting a balanced intake, focus on variety in your food choices. Incorporate diverse protein sources like legumes, nuts, and seeds while also including fortified dairy alternatives for calcium and vitamin D. Regularly reassessing your dietary choices can help identify gaps in your nutrient intake, ensuring a more comprehensive approach to nutrition.

Importance of Whole Foods vs. Processed Gluten-Free Products

Whole foods are the cornerstone of a healthy gluten-free diet. They provide essential nutrients without the additives and preservatives often found in processed gluten-free products. Opting for foods like fresh fruits, vegetables, lean proteins, and whole grains can enhance overall health and provide the necessary vitamins and minerals.

In contrast, many processed gluten-free options can be high in sugar, unhealthy fats, and low in fiber, which may negatively impact your health. To prioritize your well-being, focus on creating meals from whole foods and reserve processed alternatives for occasional treats, ensuring a healthier and more balanced diet.

Incorporating Fruits and Vegetables into Your Diet

Fruits and vegetables are vital for anyone following a gluten-free diet, providing necessary vitamins, minerals, and antioxidants. Aim to fill half your plate with a variety of colorful fruits and vegetables at each meal. Fresh, frozen, or dried options all count; just be mindful of added sugars or preservatives in processed versions.

To make it easier, consider meal prepping by washing and cutting fruits and vegetables ahead of time. This way, they are readily available for snacks or as part of a meal, promoting healthy eating habits. Try incorporating them into smoothies, salads, or as side dishes to maximize your intake and enjoy the diverse flavors they offer.

The Role of Protein Sources in a Gluten-Free Diet

Adequate protein intake is essential for maintaining muscle mass and overall health, especially on a gluten-free diet. Incorporate a variety of gluten-free protein sources, such as lean meats, fish, eggs, dairy, beans, lentils, and nuts, to meet your daily needs. Aim for protein at every meal to help stabilize blood sugar levels and promote satiety.

For those who follow a vegetarian or vegan diet, combining different plant-based protein sources, such as quinoa with black beans or chickpeas with rice, can provide all essential amino acids. Experimenting with diverse protein options will not only enhance your meals but also support a well-rounded gluten-free diet.

Understanding Fiber Intake and Gluten-Free Options

Fiber is crucial for digestive health, and gluten-free diets can sometimes lack sufficient fiber. To increase your fiber intake, choose whole fruits, vegetables, legumes, and gluten-free whole grains like brown rice, quinoa, and oats. Gradually increase your fiber consumption to prevent digestive discomfort while ensuring a varied and satisfying diet.

Incorporate high-fiber foods into each meal by adding fruits to breakfast, including beans in salads, or snacking on raw vegetables. This approach will help you reach the recommended daily intake of fiber, promoting digestive health and overall well-being.

Essential Vitamins and Minerals for Celiac Patients

Celiac patients may experience deficiencies in specific vitamins and minerals, such as B vitamins, vitamin D, calcium, iron, and zinc. Regularly including foods rich in these nutrients is vital for overall health. For instance, consider fortified gluten-free cereals for B vitamins and leafy greens or dairy alternatives for calcium and vitamin D.

To maximize absorption, pair iron-rich foods like lentils or red meat with vitamin C-rich foods like citrus fruits or bell peppers. This enhances iron absorption and helps prevent deficiencies, contributing to better health management for those with celiac disease.

Importance of Hydration and Electrolyte Balance

Staying hydrated is essential, especially for individuals with celiac disease who may experience gastrointestinal symptoms affecting fluid balance. Aim for at least eight glasses of water a day, adjusting for activity level and climate. Incorporating hydrating foods like cucumbers, watermelon, and broth-based soups can also help maintain hydration.

Electrolyte balance is critical, particularly if you experience diarrhea or vomiting. Consider electrolyte-rich beverages or homemade drinks with water, a pinch of salt, and a splash of lemon juice to replenish lost minerals. Monitoring hydration levels can ensure optimal health and support your body's functions effectively.

Recognizing Symptoms of Nutrient Deficiencies

Being aware of nutrient deficiencies is crucial for managing celiac disease effectively. Symptoms may include fatigue, weakness, brittle nails, hair loss, and frequent infections. Regularly assessing your health and consulting with a healthcare professional can help identify any deficiencies early.

If you suspect a deficiency, consider keeping a food diary to track your intake and symptoms. This practice can provide valuable insights into your nutritional habits, making it easier to identify areas for improvement and take proactive steps toward better health.

Strategies for Maintaining a Balanced Diet

To maintain a balanced diet on a gluten-free plan, focus on variety and nutrient density. Incorporate a wide range of food groups, including fruits, vegetables, whole grains, lean proteins, and healthy fats, to ensure you're meeting all your nutritional needs. Meal planning and preparation can help you avoid the temptation of gluten-containing foods.

Experiment with new recipes and gluten-free alternatives to keep your meals exciting and flavorful. Using herbs and spices can enhance taste without compromising your dietary restrictions, ensuring that you enjoy a diverse and satisfying gluten-free lifestyle.

Importance of Consulting with a Dietitian

Consulting with a registered dietitian can provide personalized guidance and support for managing a gluten-free diet. They can help assess your current dietary habits, identify nutrient deficiencies, and create a balanced meal plan tailored to your individual needs. This professional advice is particularly valuable for beginners navigating the complexities of gluten-free eating.

Dietitians can also offer practical strategies for grocery shopping, meal preparation, and dining out safely, empowering you to make informed choices. Their expertise can make the transition to a gluten-free lifestyle smoother and more sustainable, helping you achieve optimal health.

Supplements: When and What to Consider

Supplements can play a vital role in addressing nutrient deficiencies common in gluten-free diets. If you struggle to obtain adequate vitamins and minerals through food, consider consulting with a healthcare provider about potential supplements. Common options include multivitamins, calcium, vitamin D, and iron.

When choosing supplements, look for those labeled gluten-free and consider the dosage and potential interactions with any medications you may be taking. Regularly reassessing your nutritional status can help you determine whether supplements are necessary for maintaining your health.

Adapting Recipes to Boost Nutritional Value

Adapting recipes is an effective way to enhance the nutritional value of your meals while maintaining gluten-free guidelines. Start by substituting gluten-containing ingredients with whole food alternatives, such as using almond flour instead of regular flour or coconut milk instead of cream. This approach not only keeps your meals gluten-free but also boosts their nutrient content.

Incorporate nutrient-dense foods like seeds, nuts, and vegetables into your favorite recipes. For example, add chia seeds to smoothies or spinach to pasta dishes to increase fiber and vitamin intake. These simple modifications can make a significant difference in your overall nutrition while enjoying your favorite meals.

Tracking Your Nutrition for Optimal Health

Tracking your nutrition can be a valuable tool for maintaining a balanced gluten-free diet. Use apps or food journals to log your daily intake, helping you identify patterns, nutrient gaps, and areas for improvement. This awareness can empower you to make informed dietary choices and ensure you're meeting your nutritional needs.

Consider setting specific health goals, such as increasing your vegetable intake or ensuring adequate protein consumption. Regularly reviewing your tracked data can motivate you to stay on track and make adjustments as necessary, ultimately supporting your long-term health and well-being.

CHAPTER 4:

Cooking and Baking Gluten-Free

Essential Gluten-Free Cooking Techniques

To cook gluten-free effectively, begin by familiarizing yourself with your kitchen tools and appliances. Use separate cutting boards, utensils, and baking pans to avoid cross-contamination with gluten-containing foods. Always read labels on pre-packaged items, ensuring they are certified gluten-free, and clean your work surfaces thoroughly before cooking.

When preparing gluten-free meals, consider utilizing moist cooking methods, such as steaming or sautéing, which help enhance the flavor and texture of gluten-free ingredients. Experimenting with marinating proteins and using flavorful herbs and spices can elevate your dishes while keeping them safe for those with celiac disease.

Best Gluten-Free Flours and Their Uses

Understanding the various gluten-free flours available can transform your cooking. Common options include almond flour, coconut flour, and rice flour. Each flour has unique properties and is best suited for specific recipes: almond flour is great for baking, coconut flour works well in pancakes, and rice flour is ideal for creating gluten-free pasta.

To achieve the best results in baking, you can create a gluten-free flour blend by combining these flours with starches like potato or tapioca starch. This blend mimics the structure and texture of wheat flour, ensuring that your baked goods are light and fluffy.

Understanding Xanthan Gum and Its Role in Gluten-Free Baking

Xanthan gum is a crucial ingredient in gluten-free baking, acting as a binding agent that mimics gluten's elasticity. To incorporate it into your recipes, use about

1/4 to 1/2 teaspoon per cup of gluten-free flour. This will help provide structure to your baked goods, making them less crumbly and improving their overall texture.

When baking, mix xanthan gum thoroughly with your dry ingredients to ensure even distribution. This simple step can make a significant difference, allowing you to enjoy delicious, gluten-free cakes, cookies, and breads without compromising on taste or texture.

Adapting Traditional Recipes to Gluten-Free

Adapting your favorite traditional recipes to be gluten-free can be straightforward. Start by replacing all-purpose flour with a gluten-free flour blend. Be mindful that gluten-free flours often require different ratios, so it may take some trial and error to find the right measurements for your specific recipe.

In addition to changing the flour, consider the role of moisture in your dish. Gluten-free recipes may require additional liquid or binding agents like eggs to achieve the desired consistency. Taste-test your adaptations to ensure they still deliver the flavor and texture you love.

Tips for Cooking Gluten-Free Grains

Cooking gluten-free grains such as quinoa, rice, and millet is simple with a few key tips. First, rinse the grains thoroughly under cold water to remove any residue and improve flavor. Follow the package instructions for water-to-grain ratios, but a general rule is to use 2 cups of water for every cup of grains.

To enhance the taste, consider toasting grains in a dry skillet before cooking. This technique adds a nutty flavor and can elevate your meals. Once cooked, fluff the grains with a fork and incorporate them into salads, stir-fries, or as a side dish.

Common Gluten-Free Baking Mistakes to Avoid

Avoiding common mistakes in gluten-free baking can lead to better outcomes. One frequent error is not measuring ingredients accurately. Gluten-free flours vary in density, so using a scale for precision can ensure consistent results in your baking.

Another common pitfall is not allowing baked goods to cool completely before slicing. Gluten-free items often need more time to set, and cutting them too soon can result in a gummy texture. Patience is key to achieving the best results with gluten-free recipes.

Creative Uses for Gluten-Free Ingredients

Explore creative ways to incorporate gluten-free ingredients into your cooking. For example, use cauliflower rice as a low-carb substitute for traditional rice in stir-fries or grain bowls. Additionally, chickpea flour can serve as a base for making pancakes or flatbreads, adding a unique flavor profile to your meals.

Think outside the box by using nut butters or avocado as substitutes for traditional spreads on toast. This not only caters to gluten-free diets but also adds nutritional benefits and flavor diversity to your meals.

Meal Prep Ideas for Busy Lifestyles

Meal prepping can simplify your gluten-free lifestyle. Start by planning your week's meals and snacks, focusing on easy-to-cook dishes like stir-fries, soups, or salads. Prepare larger portions of grains and proteins that can be easily mixed and matched throughout the week.

Store meals in clear, labeled containers for quick access. Consider incorporating a variety of colorful vegetables and healthy fats to keep your meals balanced and appealing. This approach not only saves time but also ensures you have nutritious options readily available.

Freezing and Storing Gluten-Free Meals

Freezing gluten-free meals can help you manage your time and minimize waste. Allow cooked meals to cool completely before transferring them to airtight containers or freezer bags. Label each item with the date and contents for easy identification when you're ready to eat.

When reheating frozen meals, use a microwave or stovetop to ensure even heating. Add a splash of water to retain moisture and prevent dryness. This way, you can enjoy flavorful, home-cooked gluten-free dishes even on your busiest days.

Simple Gluten-Free Snack Ideas

Snacking gluten-free can be both delicious and straightforward. Consider whole fruits, yogurt, and nuts as quick options that require no preparation. For a bit more effort, make energy balls using gluten-free oats, nut butter, and honey, which can be stored for easy grab-and-go snacks.

Vegetable sticks paired with hummus or guacamole also make for satisfying snacks. By keeping your pantry stocked with gluten-free options, you can easily satisfy cravings without feeling restricted by your dietary needs.

Cooking for Special Occasions and Gatherings

When hosting special occasions, planning gluten-free meals can impress your guests while keeping everyone safe. Focus on naturally gluten-free dishes like roasted meats, salads, and vegetable sides. Offer a variety of options to cater to different tastes and dietary preferences.

For dessert, consider making gluten-free treats like flourless chocolate cake or gluten-free cookies. With a little creativity and planning, you can create an inclusive menu that delights all your guests, proving that gluten-free can be both festive and delicious.

Family-Friendly Gluten-Free Meals

Preparing family-friendly gluten-free meals doesn't have to be challenging. Start with simple recipes that the whole family can enjoy, like gluten-free pizza using a cauliflower crust or homemade tacos with corn tortillas. Involve your family in the cooking process to make it a fun and educational experience.

Make use of familiar flavors and textures to ease the transition. For example, serve gluten-free pasta with favorite sauces and proteins. This approach ensures that everyone, including picky eaters, can enjoy gluten-free meals without feeling deprived.

Resources for Gluten-Free Recipes and Inspiration

To explore gluten-free cooking further, numerous resources are available to guide you. Websites and blogs dedicated to gluten-free recipes can offer inspiration and new ideas. Social media platforms also feature communities where you can share experiences and find tips from others who live gluten-free.

Cookbooks focused on gluten-free diets can serve as excellent references for creating balanced meals. Libraries and online bookstores often have extensive selections that can help you expand your culinary skills and keep your meals exciting and diverse.

Chapter 5:

Dining Out and Social Situations

How to Communicate Dietary Needs to Restaurant Staff

When dining out, it's crucial to communicate your dietary needs clearly to restaurant staff. Begin by informing the host or server as soon as you arrive about your celiac disease and the necessity for a strict gluten-free meal. You can use simple phrases like, "I have celiac disease and must avoid gluten entirely. Can you help me with gluten-free options?" This direct approach ensures they understand the seriousness of your condition.

Consider having a list of gluten-free terms and dishes handy. Mention specific gluten-free options you're familiar with or inquire if the restaurant can accommodate your needs. Always ask questions about how food is prepared, as cooking methods can sometimes introduce gluten. By establishing clear communication, you create a better dining experience for yourself and increase awareness about gluten sensitivity.

Finding Gluten-Free Restaurants and Eateries

Finding gluten-free restaurants can significantly enhance your dining experience. Use online resources and apps specifically designed to locate gluten-free eateries in your area, such as Find Me Gluten Free or Gluten-Free Registry. You can also explore social media groups or local celiac support networks where members share their favorite spots. These platforms often provide reviews and feedback from others with similar dietary restrictions.

Additionally, look for restaurants that offer gluten-free menus or are certified gluten-free. Many establishments are now becoming more aware of celiac disease and offer dedicated gluten-free sections. When you call ahead, confirm their commitment to gluten-free practices, which can help you enjoy a safe meal without concerns.

Tips for Safe Dining Out with Celiac Disease

To ensure a safe dining experience, always choose restaurants that understand celiac disease and gluten-free protocols. Before visiting, review their menu online and look for gluten-free options. When you arrive, speak to the manager or chef if possible to explain your dietary needs, which will ensure they take extra precautions with your meal preparation.

When ordering, request that your meal be prepared separately from gluten-containing items and served on clean dishes. Avoid foods that could be cross-contaminated, such as fried items in shared oil. Taking these steps can help you enjoy your meal safely and reduce anxiety about dining out.

Navigating Food Allergies and Gluten-Free Menus

When faced with food allergies alongside celiac disease, it's vital to be meticulous about menu selections. Begin by informing the restaurant staff about all your dietary restrictions, as cross-contamination can occur not only with gluten but also with other allergens. This transparency helps staff understand your needs and prepare your meal safely.

In addition, seek out restaurants that explicitly cater to food allergies and gluten-free diets. Many establishments now highlight their gluten-free options and allergen-free menus. Make sure to ask how dishes are prepared and if the ingredients are free from gluten and allergens, ensuring a safe and enjoyable dining experience.

Preparing for Social Events: What to Bring

When attending social events, preparation is key to ensuring you can safely enjoy the food. Consider bringing your own gluten-free dish or snacks to share, which can help ease your worries about gluten exposure. When hosting, make sure to inform the host about your dietary needs in advance, so they can provide safe options.

Additionally, consider packing gluten-free snacks in case there are limited options at the event. Foods like fruit, nuts, or gluten-free granola bars can keep you satisfied while allowing you to participate in socializing without feeling left out or anxious about your dietary needs.

Handling Peer Pressure and Social Situations

Dealing with peer pressure regarding your dietary choices can be challenging. It's essential to be firm yet polite when explaining your condition to friends. A simple, "I have celiac disease, so I can't eat gluten," can help your peers understand why you need to stick to your dietary restrictions without feeling uncomfortable.

Surround yourself with supportive friends who respect your choices. If you're in a situation where gluten is present, focus on enjoying your company rather than the food. Having a plan, such as bringing your own gluten-free snacks, can also alleviate pressure and ensure you feel included without compromising your health.

Understanding Cross-Contamination in Restaurants

Cross-contamination is a significant concern for those with celiac disease. Understanding how it occurs can help you navigate dining out more safely. This can happen when gluten-free foods come into contact with gluten-containing items, such as shared utensils, cutting boards, or cooking surfaces. Always inquire about food preparation processes to minimize risks.

Educating yourself about common cross-contamination practices allows you to ask the right questions at restaurants. For example, ask if they use separate frying oil for gluten-free items or if they have dedicated equipment for gluten-free food preparation. Understanding these details will empower you to make safer dining choices.

Strategies for Eating Out While Traveling

When traveling, maintaining a gluten-free diet requires a little planning. Start by researching gluten-free options in the area you'll be visiting. Apps and websites can help you locate suitable restaurants, and many travel blogs offer tips for dining gluten-free in specific cities. Make a list of places to try ahead of time.

Pack gluten-free snacks to have on hand while exploring new places, as finding suitable meals may take time. Additionally, consider accommodations with kitchen facilities, allowing you to prepare some meals yourself. By preparing in advance, you can enjoy your trip without stressing about food choices.

Educating Friends and Family about Celiac Disease

Informing your friends and family about celiac disease is essential for building a supportive environment. Start by explaining what celiac disease is, emphasizing that it's an autoimmune disorder and not just a dietary preference. Share how gluten affects your health and the importance of avoiding cross-contamination.

Encourage open dialogue by inviting them to ask questions and express their concerns. Provide them with resources, such as pamphlets or websites, to help them understand better. This knowledge helps foster an understanding that leads to greater support when socializing or dining together.

Importance of Planning Ahead for Meals

Planning meals in advance is crucial for managing celiac disease effectively. Take time each week to create a meal plan that includes gluten-free recipes and ingredients. This proactive approach helps you avoid last-minute decisions that could lead to unsafe food choices.

When grocery shopping, stick to your meal plan and look for gluten-free labels on products. Preparing meals in batches can also save time during busy weeks. By having gluten-free meals readily available, you reduce the risk of exposure and ensure you're meeting your dietary needs consistently.

Dealing with Well-Meaning but Uninformed Friends

Well-meaning friends may unintentionally cause stress by offering gluten-containing foods or making suggestions that aren't safe. Approach these situations with kindness and education. When a friend offers you food, politely decline and explain your dietary restrictions. This fosters understanding rather than resentment.

Consider providing gluten-free alternatives during gatherings to demonstrate that safe options can be delicious. Sharing your experiences with celiac disease can help friends learn and adjust their behaviors over time. Their willingness to understand your needs is essential in maintaining your relationships and ensuring your safety.

Embracing Social Situations with Confidence

Embracing social situations is vital for maintaining a balanced lifestyle with celiac disease. Prepare yourself by familiarizing yourself with gluten-free options at venues before attending events. Confidence in your dietary choices can help you enjoy social gatherings without anxiety about food.

Practice assertiveness when discussing your needs. Clear communication with hosts and friends about your dietary restrictions fosters understanding and support. Embracing your condition with confidence allows you to focus on the social aspects of gatherings rather than worrying about food safety.

Finding Support During Social Gatherings

Finding support in social situations can make managing celiac disease easier. If possible, connect with fellow celiac individuals at events. Having someone who understands your dietary restrictions can create a sense of camaraderie and ease during meals.

Don't hesitate to communicate with the host or event planner about your needs ahead of time. This proactive approach can lead to accommodations, such as gluten-free options. Joining support groups or online communities can also provide valuable resources and encouragement, helping you feel more connected and supported in your gluten-free journey.

CHAPTER 6:

Managing Celiac Disease in Children

Recognizing Celiac Disease Symptoms in Children

Celiac disease symptoms in children can vary widely but commonly include digestive issues like diarrhea, bloating, and abdominal pain. Other symptoms may include fatigue, irritability, and delayed growth. Parents should be vigilant about these signs, especially if there is a family history of celiac disease or autoimmune disorders. Keeping a food diary can help identify patterns and triggers related to gluten consumption.

To effectively recognize symptoms, parents should monitor their child's reactions to different foods, particularly those containing gluten, such as wheat, barley, and rye. Regular check-ups with a pediatrician can facilitate early diagnosis, and blood tests or intestinal biopsies may be necessary for confirmation.

Understanding the symptoms early can lead to timely intervention and management.

Supporting Children through Diagnosis and Treatment

When a child is diagnosed with celiac disease, emotional support is crucial. Parents should create an open dialogue, reassuring their child that the diagnosis is manageable and not their fault. Educating the child about celiac disease, its implications, and the importance of a gluten-free diet can empower them and reduce feelings of anxiety or isolation.

Treatment primarily involves adhering to a strict gluten-free diet. Parents should work with healthcare providers or nutritionists to create a balanced diet plan, ensuring their child receives all necessary nutrients. Regular follow-ups can help track progress and make dietary adjustments as needed, providing ongoing support and encouragement.

Navigating School Lunches and Activities

To ensure a safe and enjoyable school experience for children with celiac disease, it's essential to communicate with school staff. Parents should discuss their child's dietary restrictions with teachers, cafeteria staff, and school nurses, ensuring they understand the need for gluten-free options and avoiding cross-contamination during meal preparation.

Preparing gluten-free lunchboxes can make lunchtime stress-free. Parents can pack nutritious and appealing meals, such as gluten-free wraps, fruits, and vegetables, allowing children to enjoy their meals alongside peers. Encouraging children to bring their gluten-free snacks for parties and activities can foster inclusivity and minimize feelings of exclusion during school events.

Gluten-Free Snacks for Kids on-the-Go

Busy lifestyles can make it challenging to find gluten-free snacks for kids. Parents can prepare easy, on-the-go options like gluten-free granola bars, rice cakes, or fruit and nut mixes. Having a stash of these snacks at home and in the car ensures kids always have something safe to eat, preventing hunger-related meltdowns.

Teaching children to choose gluten-free snacks themselves can encourage independence and make snack time enjoyable. Stores often carry gluten-free products, so involving kids in shopping can be fun and educational. Parents can guide their children on how to read labels and identify safe snacks, helping them make informed choices.

Encouraging Healthy Eating Habits

Promoting healthy eating habits is essential for children with celiac disease. Parents should emphasize whole, unprocessed foods like fruits, vegetables, lean proteins, and gluten-free grains such as quinoa and rice.

Involving children in meal preparation can make healthy eating more appealing and teach them valuable cooking skills.

Setting a positive example is key; when parents maintain a healthy diet, children are more likely to follow suit. Regular family meals can reinforce good eating habits, providing a structured environment where healthy choices are the norm. Encouraging mindful eating, where children pay attention to hunger cues and enjoy their food, can further enhance their relationship with food.

Teaching Children About Food Choices and Safety

Educating children about food choices is vital in managing celiac disease. Parents should explain what gluten is, where it is found, and why avoiding it is essential for their health. Creating a simple visual guide or using apps to help children identify safe and unsafe foods can make learning engaging and interactive.

Safety is paramount when it comes to food. Parents should teach children to ask questions about food preparation when dining out or at friends' houses. Encouraging them to speak up about their dietary restrictions fosters confidence and ensures they can navigate food situations independently as they grow.

Planning Birthday Parties and Celebrations

Planning birthday parties for children with celiac disease can be challenging but manageable. Parents should communicate with other parents about gluten-free cake and snack options and ensure safe food is available for their child. Using gluten-free recipes for treats can also ensure that everyone at the party can enjoy the food without concerns.

Incorporating gluten-free activities, like decorating cookies or cupcakes, can make celebrations fun and inclusive. Providing a variety of gluten-free options can help all guests feel included, allowing the birthday child to celebrate without feeling left out. Creating a gluten-free party menu not only supports the child but also educates other kids about dietary restrictions.

Building a Support System for Parents

Creating a support network can significantly ease the challenges of managing a child's celiac disease. Parents should connect with other families who have children with celiac disease, either through local support groups or online communities. Sharing experiences, recipes, and tips can provide encouragement and practical advice.

Building relationships with healthcare professionals, including dietitians and pediatricians, is also crucial. These experts can offer guidance and reassurance, helping parents navigate the complexities of a gluten-free lifestyle. Establishing a solid support system empowers parents to advocate effectively for their children's health and well-being.

Understanding the Emotional Impact on Children

Children with celiac disease may experience a range of emotions, including frustration, sadness, or anxiety related to their dietary restrictions. It's essential for parents to recognize and validate these feelings, fostering an environment where children feel safe to express themselves. Open communication about their feelings can help children process their emotions and build resilience.

Involving children in the management of their condition can empower them and reduce feelings of helplessness. Encouraging participation in meal planning and cooking, as well as discussing experiences with peers, can help them feel more in control. Parents should also remain vigilant about potential bullying or teasing, ensuring their child has coping strategies and support when faced with challenges.

Resources for Child-Friendly Gluten-Free Meals

Numerous resources are available to assist parents in finding child-friendly gluten-free meal options. Websites and cookbooks dedicated to gluten-free cooking can provide inspiration and practical recipes. Utilizing meal planning apps that cater to gluten-free diets can simplify grocery shopping and meal preparation.

Local grocery stores often have gluten-free sections, and many brands now offer kid-friendly products. Parents should explore options like gluten-free pasta, cereals, and snacks, making it easier to create familiar meals that children enjoy. Joining gluten-free forums or social media groups can also provide additional ideas and support from other parents.

Discussing Celiac Disease with Peers

Teaching children how to discuss their celiac disease with peers is an essential life skill. Parents can role-play conversations to help children feel more comfortable explaining their condition and dietary needs. Emphasizing that celiac disease is a medical condition, not a choice, can help peers understand and support their friend.

Encouraging open dialogue fosters empathy among peers. Parents can provide children with simple explanations to share with friends, enabling them to communicate their needs effectively. This approach not only builds understanding but also helps reduce the stigma surrounding dietary restrictions.

Tips for Adjusting Family Meals for Children

When adjusting family meals to accommodate a child with celiac disease, parents should prioritize gluten-free substitutions for favorite dishes. Instead of traditional pasta, consider using gluten-free alternatives made from rice or corn. Making small changes, like gluten-free breadcrumbs or flour, allows families to enjoy meals together without sacrificing taste.

Planning family meals that are naturally gluten-free, such as grilled meats, vegetables, and salads, can simplify meal preparation. Engaging children in choosing meals can also make them feel more involved and excited about food. Keeping family favorites adaptable ensures everyone enjoys mealtime without stress.

Keeping Up with Dietary Changes as Children Grow

As children grow, their dietary needs and preferences may evolve. Parents should remain attentive to their child's nutritional requirements, ensuring they receive a balanced diet rich in vitamins and minerals. Regular check-ins with healthcare providers can help monitor growth and development while addressing any emerging dietary concerns.

Adapting to dietary changes may involve trying new gluten-free foods or exploring different cooking methods. Encouraging children to participate in grocery shopping and cooking fosters independence and helps them develop a positive relationship with food. Keeping the lines of communication open about their preferences allows families to adapt meals while ensuring they remain gluten-free.

CHAPTER 7:

Coping with the Emotional Aspects of Celiac Disease

Understanding the Psychological Impact of Celiac Disease

Celiac disease not only affects physical health but can also significantly impact mental well-being. The diagnosis often brings feelings of anxiety and fear regarding food choices, social situations, and potential health repercussions. Understanding these psychological effects is essential for developing coping strategies. Acknowledging that emotional reactions are normal can help individuals process their feelings, leading to better management of their health.

It's vital to recognize that the stress of navigating a gluten-free lifestyle can be overwhelming. Many experience a sense of loss over their previous eating habits or feel isolated due to dietary restrictions. Seeking education about the disease and its implications can empower individuals to take control of their situation, fostering a healthier mental outlook.

Managing Anxiety Around Food and Eating

Anxiety about food is common among those with celiac disease, especially when dining out or attending social gatherings. Preparing in advance can help mitigate these feelings. Start by researching restaurant menus beforehand or packing your own gluten-free snacks for outings. Familiarizing yourself with safe food options can ease anxiety and help you feel more in control.

Practicing mindful eating can also help reduce food-related anxiety. This involves focusing on the flavors and textures of your food, as well as appreciating each meal. Mindfulness techniques, such as deep breathing before meals, can help ground you and promote a positive eating experience, transforming the act of eating from a source of stress into a moment of enjoyment.

Building a Positive Relationship with Food

A positive relationship with food is crucial for long-term health and well-being. This involves shifting your focus from what you cannot eat to the diverse array of gluten-free foods available. Explore new recipes and ingredients to discover meals that excite and nourish you. Engaging in the culinary process can foster enjoyment and creativity, turning cooking into a therapeutic experience.

Additionally, practicing gratitude for the meals you can enjoy can help reshape your mindset. Instead of viewing gluten-free eating as a restriction, see it as an opportunity to nourish your body in new ways. Emphasizing enjoyment and variety in your diet can lead to a more fulfilling relationship with food.

Strategies for Coping with Frustration and Isolation

Coping with frustration and feelings of isolation is an important aspect of managing celiac disease. One effective strategy is to maintain a journal where you can express your feelings and experiences. Writing can provide a safe space to process your emotions and reflect on your gluten-free journey. It can also help track challenges and identify patterns that may need addressing.

Engaging in open conversations with family and friends about your feelings can also alleviate isolation. Sharing your experiences and struggles can foster understanding and support from loved ones. Building these connections not only combats loneliness but also reinforces your support system, helping you feel less alone in your journey.

Finding Community and Support Networks

Connecting with others who share similar experiences can provide invaluable support. Look for local or online support groups focused on celiac disease or gluten sensitivity. These communities offer a platform for sharing resources, recipes, and coping strategies, helping you feel connected to others facing similar challenges.

Additionally, social media can be a powerful tool for finding support. Follow gluten-free bloggers and join relevant groups to access a wealth of information and community. Engaging with these networks can provide motivation, encouragement, and a sense of belonging, enhancing your overall well-being.

Mindfulness and Its Benefits for Emotional Health

Incorporating mindfulness into your daily routine can significantly improve emotional health. Mindfulness involves being present in the moment and acknowledging your thoughts and feelings without judgment. Simple practices like meditation or deep-breathing exercises can help reduce stress and anxiety associated with managing celiac disease.

To integrate mindfulness into your life, start with a few minutes of focused breathing each day. Gradually extend this time as you become more comfortable. You can also practice mindfulness during meals by savoring each bite and appreciating the nourishment it provides. This practice can help you cultivate a deeper connection with food and enhance your emotional resilience.

Recognizing Signs of Depression or Anxiety

Being aware of the signs of depression or anxiety is crucial for maintaining mental health when living with celiac disease. Common symptoms include persistent sadness, withdrawal from social activities, changes in appetite, and feelings of hopelessness. Regular self-check-ins can help you recognize these signs early and seek appropriate help if needed.

If you notice these signs, consider reaching out to a mental health professional for support. They can provide coping strategies and techniques tailored to your needs. Early intervention is key to managing these symptoms effectively and ensuring they do not hinder your ability to enjoy life.

The Importance of Self-Advocacy

Self-advocacy is essential for managing celiac disease effectively. This involves being proactive about your health needs, including communicating your dietary restrictions to family, friends, and restaurant staff. Don't hesitate to ask questions or request modifications to meals to ensure your safety and comfort.

Additionally, educating yourself about celiac disease empowers you to advocate for your health. Understanding your rights, such as the legal protections regarding food labeling, can help you navigate situations confidently. Self-advocacy fosters a sense of control and can significantly enhance your overall experience with celiac disease.

Celebrating Small Victories in the Gluten-Free Journey

Recognizing and celebrating small victories can enhance your motivation and positivity throughout your gluten-free journey. These victories can include trying a new recipe, successfully navigating a social event, or simply feeling well after a meal. Taking time to acknowledge these moments reinforces the progress you're making and boosts your confidence.

Consider keeping a victory journal where you document these achievements. Reflecting on your progress can provide encouragement during challenging times. Celebrating even the smallest successes can cultivate a positive mindset and foster resilience in your gluten-free lifestyle.

Maintaining a Positive Mindset

A positive mindset is crucial for managing celiac disease and navigating its challenges. Start by cultivating gratitude and focusing on what you can enjoy rather than what you can't. This shift in perspective can help you appreciate your gluten-free meals and the vibrant, nourishing foods available to you.

Incorporating positive affirmations into your daily routine can also be beneficial. Repeating phrases that reinforce your strength and resilience can help combat negative thoughts. Surrounding yourself with supportive individuals and engaging in activities that bring you joy can further enhance your positive outlook.

Engaging in Stress-Relief Activities

Finding effective stress-relief activities can significantly improve your emotional well-being while managing celiac disease. Activities such as yoga, walking in nature, or engaging in a creative hobby can help alleviate stress and promote relaxation. Identify activities that resonate with you and incorporate them into your routine.

Establishing a regular practice of stress relief can enhance your resilience in the face of challenges. Schedule dedicated time each week for these activities, treating them as essential self-care. By prioritizing your mental health, you equip yourself to better handle the stresses of living with celiac disease.

Balancing Life Beyond Celiac Disease

Celiac disease is just one aspect of your life, and finding balance is essential for overall well-being. Engaging in hobbies, social activities, and personal interests outside of your dietary restrictions can promote a fulfilling life. Make time for activities that excite you and allow you to connect with others, creating a well-rounded lifestyle.

Creating a schedule that includes both gluten-free meal planning and time for social engagements can help maintain this balance. Prioritize self-care and ensure you allocate time for relaxation and enjoyment. By nurturing all areas of your life, you can foster a holistic approach to managing celiac disease.

Seeking Professional Help If Needed

Recognizing when to seek professional help is crucial for maintaining your mental health while managing celiac disease. If feelings of depression or anxiety become overwhelming, consulting with a mental health professional can provide valuable support. Therapy can offer coping strategies tailored to your specific experiences, helping you navigate challenges more effectively.

Additionally, consider reaching out to a registered dietitian who specializes in celiac disease for nutritional guidance. They can help you create a balanced gluten-free meal plan, ensuring you meet your dietary needs. Professional support can be instrumental in managing both the physical and emotional aspects of living with celiac disease.

CHAPTER 8:

Staying Informed and Engaged

Importance of Ongoing Education about Celiac Disease

Ongoing education about celiac disease is crucial for effectively managing the condition and avoiding health complications. Understanding the autoimmune nature of celiac disease, its symptoms, and the importance of a strict gluten-free diet helps individuals make informed decisions about their health. This includes learning about potential cross-contamination, hidden sources of gluten, and how to read food labels accurately. By continually seeking knowledge, individuals can better navigate their dietary restrictions and enhance their overall well-being.

Additionally, education helps individuals stay aware of potential health risks associated with untreated celiac disease, such as malnutrition and other autoimmune disorders. Educational resources include reputable websites, books, and workshops focused on celiac disease. Participating in educational sessions not only equips individuals with necessary skills but also fosters a supportive network of peers who share similar experiences.

Latest Research and Developments in Celiac Disease

Staying informed about the latest research and developments in celiac disease is essential for anyone affected by this condition. New studies may offer insights into the genetic factors that contribute to celiac disease, as well as advancements in potential treatments and therapies. Understanding these findings can empower individuals to engage in informed discussions with healthcare providers and make decisions that best support their health.

Additionally, research continues to improve gluten detection methods and alternative treatments, such as enzyme therapies that may aid gluten digestion. Following reputable medical journals and organizations specializing in celiac disease can help individuals stay updated on these developments and consider emerging options in their management plans.

Joining Celiac Disease Advocacy Organizations

Joining celiac disease advocacy organizations can provide valuable resources and support for individuals navigating this condition. These organizations often offer educational materials, community events, and access to the latest research and developments in celiac disease management. Becoming a member can also connect individuals with others facing similar challenges, creating a sense of belonging and shared experience.

Additionally, advocacy groups work to raise awareness and promote policy changes that improve access to gluten-free products and labeling. Participating in these organizations can enhance one's voice in the community and contribute to broader efforts aimed at improving the quality of life for those with celiac disease.

Engaging with Gluten-Free Communities Online

Engaging with gluten-free communities online is a practical way to share experiences and gain insights from others who understand the challenges of living with celiac disease. Many forums and social media groups provide a platform to ask questions, share recipes, and discuss coping strategies. By actively participating in these communities, individuals can learn from the successes and setbacks of others, making their own gluten-free journey more manageable.

Moreover, these online communities often highlight new gluten-free products and restaurants, allowing individuals to discover safe dining options and innovative meal ideas. Being part of an online network can foster a sense of camaraderie and support, providing encouragement during difficult times.

Staying Updated on Gluten-Free Products

Staying updated on gluten-free products is essential for managing celiac disease effectively. Regularly checking product labels and researching new gluten-free items can help individuals find safe alternatives to their favorite foods. Many brands are continuously expanding their gluten-free offerings, and staying informed about these changes ensures that individuals have access to a variety of safe and delicious options.

Additionally, utilizing apps and websites dedicated to gluten-free product listings can streamline this process. These tools often include user reviews, safety ratings, and tips for finding gluten-free options at local stores. By actively seeking out and trying new products, individuals can enhance their gluten-free lifestyle and prevent dietary monotony.

Understanding the Role of Social Media in Celiac Support

Social media plays a significant role in providing support for individuals with celiac disease. Platforms like Instagram, Facebook, and Twitter allow users to connect with influencers, dietitians, and fellow celiac warriors who share tips, recipes, and personal stories. By following relevant accounts, individuals can access a wealth of information and support while also contributing their own experiences to the community.

Moreover, social media can raise awareness about celiac disease and its impact on daily life, helping to destigmatize the condition. Sharing posts and participating in discussions can foster understanding among friends and family, creating a more supportive environment for those managing celiac disease.

Following Blogs and Podcasts on Gluten-Free Living

Following blogs and podcasts dedicated to gluten-free living can provide ongoing inspiration and practical advice for those with celiac disease. Many bloggers and podcasters share personal stories, cooking tips, and product recommendations, making the gluten-free lifestyle more accessible and enjoyable. Engaging with this content can also offer insight into the latest research and developments in the field.

Additionally, these platforms often feature guest experts, such as dietitians and chefs, who provide valuable information on maintaining a balanced diet while avoiding gluten. By incorporating insights from blogs and podcasts into their daily lives, individuals can enhance their understanding of celiac disease and feel more empowered in their dietary choices.

Participating in Gluten-Free Events and Expos

Participating in gluten-free events and expos can be a fun and educational way to immerse oneself in the gluten-free community. These gatherings often feature vendors showcasing gluten-free products, cooking demonstrations, and informative sessions led by health professionals. Attending such events allows individuals to discover new products, learn cooking techniques, and connect with others who share similar dietary needs.

Moreover, these events often provide opportunities to ask questions and seek advice from experts in the field. Engaging in discussions with manufacturers and fellow attendees can lead to valuable insights and resources that enhance one's gluten-free lifestyle.

Sharing Personal Experiences to Help Others

Sharing personal experiences can significantly impact the lives of others managing celiac disease. By recounting one's journey, challenges, and successes, individuals can provide support and encouragement to those who may be struggling. This sharing fosters a sense of community and solidarity among those facing similar obstacles, reminding them that they are not alone in their journey.

Additionally, personal stories can raise awareness about the condition and help educate others about its complexities. Whether through social media, blogs, or support groups, sharing experiences can empower others to take charge of their health and advocate for themselves.

Importance of Advocating for Gluten-Free Labeling

Advocating for gluten-free labeling is crucial for individuals with celiac disease to ensure their safety while navigating food options. Clear labeling helps consumers identify safe products, reducing the risk of accidental gluten ingestion. By supporting initiatives aimed at stricter labeling regulations, individuals can contribute to the protection of those with gluten sensitivities and celiac disease.

Moreover, raising awareness about the importance of gluten-free labeling can help educate manufacturers and retailers about the needs of consumers. This advocacy can lead to improved product transparency and an overall increase in the availability of safe gluten-free options in the market.

Building Relationships with Healthcare Providers

Building strong relationships with healthcare providers is essential for effectively managing celiac disease. Regular communication with doctors, dietitians, and specialists can help individuals receive personalized guidance on their dietary needs and health management strategies. Establishing trust allows for open discussions about symptoms, dietary challenges, and potential treatments, leading to better health outcomes.

Additionally, healthcare providers can offer referrals to specialists and support groups, further enhancing an individual's resources for managing their condition. Engaging actively with healthcare professionals can empower individuals to take charge of their health and make informed decisions about their gluten-free lifestyle.

Creating Awareness in Your Community

Creating awareness in your community about celiac disease can foster understanding and support for those affected. Organizing informational sessions, distributing pamphlets, or speaking at local events can help educate others about the condition, its symptoms, and the importance of a gluten-free diet. Increased awareness can reduce stigma and encourage individuals to seek help if they suspect they have celiac disease.

Moreover, raising awareness can lead to improved accommodations for those with dietary restrictions in schools, workplaces, and restaurants. By advocating for inclusive practices, individuals can help ensure a supportive environment for everyone managing celiac disease.

Encouraging Family and Friends to Learn About Celiac Disease

Encouraging family and friends to learn about celiac disease can create a supportive network for those affected. By sharing educational resources and personal experiences, individuals can help their loved ones understand the importance of a gluten-free diet and how to avoid gluten cross-contamination. This understanding can significantly reduce the risk of accidental gluten ingestion during family meals and social gatherings.

Additionally, fostering open conversations about dietary needs can strengthen relationships and create a more inclusive atmosphere. When family and friends are informed about celiac disease, they are better equipped to provide support and ensure that social situations are comfortable for everyone involved.

CHAPTER 9:

Conclusion and Next Steps

Recap of Key Points from the Book

In managing celiac disease, understanding gluten and its impact on health is crucial. Key points include recognizing gluten-containing foods, reading labels diligently, and being aware of cross-contamination risks. This knowledge helps prevent accidental gluten ingestion, ensuring a safe gluten-free diet. Additionally, focusing on whole foods like fruits, vegetables, meats, and gluten-free grains can create a balanced and nourishing diet that supports your overall health.

Effective management also involves understanding your body's reactions and maintaining regular health check-ups. Keeping a food diary can help identify trigger foods and monitor symptoms, enabling you to make informed choices. This recap emphasizes the importance of continuous education and adapting your lifestyle to maintain long-term health and well-being.

Encouragement to Embrace the Gluten-Free Lifestyle

Embracing a gluten-free lifestyle can feel overwhelming at first, but it can also lead to significant improvements in your health and quality of life. Start by exploring gluten-free alternatives that suit your taste preferences, such as rice, quinoa, and gluten-free flours for baking. Experimenting with new recipes can be an exciting way to enhance your culinary skills while ensuring you avoid gluten.

Social situations may also present challenges, but advocating for yourself and communicating your dietary needs can help others understand your requirements. As you grow more comfortable in your gluten-free journey, you'll find ways to enjoy meals with friends and family without compromising your health.

Strategies for Continuous Improvement and Adaptation

Continuous improvement in managing celiac disease involves regularly assessing your dietary choices and lifestyle habits. Begin by setting aside time to review your meal plans and recipes, ensuring they align with gluten-free guidelines. Incorporating new foods and techniques into your cooking can keep your meals fresh and enjoyable, making it easier to stick to your gluten-free diet.

Adapting to changes in your health or lifestyle may also require reassessing your approach. Engage with support groups or forums to share experiences and strategies with others who are navigating similar challenges. This sense of community can provide valuable insights and encouragement as you continue to refine your gluten-free lifestyle.

Resources for Ongoing Support and Education

Finding reliable resources is essential for maintaining a gluten-free lifestyle. Start by exploring websites, cookbooks, and online communities dedicated to celiac disease and gluten sensitivity. Many organizations provide valuable information, including meal plans, recipes, and tips for dining out safely. Consider subscribing to newsletters or blogs that offer new recipes and research updates related to gluten-free living.

Additionally, local support groups can offer emotional support and practical advice. Connecting with others facing similar challenges can be uplifting, providing you with a sense of belonging while sharing helpful strategies for navigating your gluten-free journey. Regularly updating your knowledge will empower you to make informed decisions for your health.

Importance of Self-Care and Personal Well-Being

Self-care is vital for those managing celiac disease, as it helps maintain mental and physical health. Incorporating activities such as mindfulness, yoga, or meditation can alleviate stress and enhance your overall well-being. Prioritize self-care by dedicating time to relax and engage in activities that bring you joy, whether it's cooking gluten-free meals or spending time with loved ones.

Regular exercise also plays a significant role in your health journey. Aim to find activities that you enjoy, as this will motivate you to stay active. Focusing on both physical and emotional well-being ensures you remain resilient as you navigate the challenges of living gluten-free.

Setting Realistic Goals for Your Gluten-Free Journey

Setting realistic goals is essential for a successful gluten-free journey. Start by identifying specific areas of your life that you want to improve, such as meal planning, grocery shopping, or trying new gluten-free recipes. Break these larger goals into smaller, manageable tasks, allowing you to track your progress without feeling overwhelmed.

As you achieve these small milestones, celebrate your successes, no matter how minor they may seem. This sense of accomplishment will motivate you to continue working toward your larger goals, fostering a positive mindset that enhances your overall gluten-free experience.

Celebrating Milestones and Achievements

Celebrating milestones in your gluten-free journey is crucial for maintaining motivation and positivity. Take the time to acknowledge your progress, whether it's mastering a new gluten-free recipe, successfully navigating a restaurant menu, or going a month without gluten-related symptoms. Share these achievements with friends and family, who can help you celebrate and provide encouragement.

Consider creating a personal journal or visual board to document your milestones. This tangible reminder of your progress can serve as a powerful motivator, reinforcing your commitment to living a gluten-free lifestyle and inspiring you to set new goals as you move forward.

Encouraging a Proactive Approach to Health

A proactive approach to health involves staying informed and making conscious choices that positively impact your well-being. Schedule regular check-ups with healthcare providers to monitor your condition and adjust your dietary plan as needed. Being proactive means anticipating potential challenges and preparing for them, such as researching gluten-free options before dining out or packing safe snacks for travel

Taking charge of your health also includes educating yourself about the latest research and developments in celiac disease management. Staying engaged with ongoing education empowers you to advocate for yourself and make informed decisions about your gluten-free lifestyle.

Building Resilience and Confidence

Building resilience and confidence in your gluten-free journey is essential for overcoming challenges. Start by acknowledging any setbacks or frustrations you encounter and treat them as learning opportunities rather than failures. Reflect on what you can change to avoid similar issues in the future, which will help you grow stronger and more adaptable.

Participating in gluten-free communities, both online and in-person, can also boost your confidence. Sharing your experiences and learning from others fosters a sense of camaraderie, reminding you that you're not alone in this journey. Over time, you'll build the resilience needed to navigate any obstacles that arise.

Keeping a Positive Outlook on Living Gluten-Free

Maintaining a positive outlook on living gluten-free can significantly enhance your experience. Focus on the benefits of a gluten-free lifestyle, such as improved health and energy levels. Surround yourself with supportive friends and family who understand your dietary needs and can help foster a positive environment.

Engage in activities that promote joy, such as cooking and exploring new gluten-free foods. By prioritizing positivity and gratitude for the healthy choices you're making, you'll find it easier to stay committed to your gluten-free lifestyle.

Ways to Inspire Others through Your Journey

Your journey to living gluten-free can inspire others to embrace healthier choices. Share your experiences through social media, blogs, or community groups, highlighting the positive aspects of your journey. Consider hosting gluten-free cooking classes or workshops to educate others about delicious, safe meal options.

Be open about your challenges and triumphs, as this authenticity can resonate with those struggling to make similar lifestyle changes. By sharing your story, you empower others to embark on their own gluten-free journeys, creating a supportive network of individuals committed to better health.

Recognizing the Long-Term Benefits of a Gluten-Free Diet

Understanding the long-term benefits of a gluten-free diet can reinforce your commitment to this lifestyle. A well-managed gluten-free diet can lead to improved digestive health, enhanced energy levels, and better nutrient absorption. Recognizing these benefits encourages you to remain diligent in avoiding gluten and prioritizing your health.

Additionally, many individuals experience increased mental clarity and reduced inflammation when adhering to a gluten-free diet. Regularly reflecting on these positive changes can help motivate you to continue making mindful choices that support your long-term health and well-being.

Commitment to Lifelong Learning and Advocacy

Commitment to lifelong learning is crucial for effectively managing celiac disease. Stay updated on research developments and dietary guidelines by reading books, articles, and attending seminars related to gluten sensitivity and celiac disease. By staying informed, you can adjust your practices and share valuable insights with others.

Advocating for yourself and others in the gluten-free community is equally important. Engage in discussions about celiac disease awareness and participate in initiatives that promote gluten-free options in restaurants and grocery stores. Your advocacy efforts can significantly impact not only your life but also the lives of many others navigating similar challenges.

Common Concerns

What if I accidentally consume gluten?

If you accidentally consume gluten, the first step is to remain calm and assess your symptoms. Many people with celiac disease experience immediate reactions, including gastrointestinal discomfort, fatigue, or skin rashes. Keep a symptom diary to track any reactions you might have, as this can help you and your healthcare provider adjust your management plan effectively.

To manage the situation, stay hydrated and rest your body. You might also consider taking over-the-counter medications for symptom relief, such as antacids or anti-diarrheal medications, after consulting with your doctor. Make a note to review your food sources and identify how the gluten exposure occurred to help prevent future accidents.

Can I outgrow celiac disease?

Celiac disease is a lifelong autoimmune condition; most individuals do not outgrow it. Once diagnosed, adhering to a strict gluten-free diet is essential to avoid damage to the small intestine and long-term health complications. While some children may exhibit symptoms that appear to lessen with age, this does not indicate an outgrown condition.

It's crucial to have regular check-ups with your healthcare provider to monitor your health status and ensure you are maintaining a gluten-free lifestyle. Continuous education about celiac disease and staying vigilant about your diet is essential to managing the condition effectively throughout your life.

How do I manage symptoms during a flare-up?

During a flare-up, focus on self-care strategies to alleviate symptoms. This may include drinking plenty of fluids, consuming bland foods such as rice, bananas, or applesauce, and avoiding dairy products, which can sometimes exacerbate symptoms. Keeping a food diary can help you identify specific triggers and patterns in your symptoms.

Additionally, rest is vital during a flare-up to allow your body to recover. You may also want to consult your healthcare provider for advice on symptom management and any appropriate medications to ease discomfort. Establishing a solid support system, such as a celiac disease support group, can also be beneficial for emotional support and practical tips

Is a gluten-free diet healthy?

A gluten-free diet can be healthy if it is well-balanced and includes a variety of whole, unprocessed foods. Focus on naturally gluten-free foods such as fruits, vegetables, lean proteins, nuts, seeds, and gluten-free grains like quinoa and brown rice. Ensure you're not solely relying on processed gluten-free products, which may be high in sugars and unhealthy fats.

To maintain a balanced diet, plan meals ahead, and incorporate various food groups. Pay attention to nutrient density, focusing on foods rich in fiber, vitamins, and minerals. Consider working with a dietitian who specializes in celiac disease to help you create a meal plan that meets your nutritional needs while being entirely gluten-free.

What are the best gluten-free grains?

The best gluten-free grains include quinoa, brown rice, millet, buckwheat, and amaranth. These grains are not only safe for individuals with celiac disease but also provide essential nutrients and fiber. Incorporating a variety of these grains into your diet helps ensure a balanced intake of carbohydrates and other nutrients.

When selecting gluten-free grains, opt for whole grains whenever possible for added health benefits. Experiment with different grains to find what you enjoy and how to incorporate them into meals—such as using quinoa in salads or brown rice as a base for stir-fries. Always check for gluten-free certifications on packaging to avoid cross-contamination.

How can I ensure I get enough nutrients?

To ensure you get enough nutrients while on a gluten-free diet, focus on a diverse and balanced diet that includes various fruits, vegetables, proteins, and gluten-free grains. Incorporating a wide range of foods helps to meet your nutritional requirements and prevent deficiencies.

Consider taking gluten-free multivitamins or specific supplements, such as iron, calcium, and vitamin D, especially if you struggle to meet your needs through diet alone. Consulting with a healthcare provider or dietitian can help assess your nutrient intake and recommend tailored supplementation if necessary.

Are gluten-free processed foods safe?

Gluten-free processed foods can be safe for individuals with celiac disease, but caution is essential. Always check labels for gluten-free certifications and be aware of potential cross-contamination during processing. Some gluten-free processed foods may contain additives or ingredients that are not nutrient-dense, so read the nutritional information carefully.

Limit your intake of processed gluten-free foods, as they can be high in sugars, unhealthy fats, and low in fiber. Aim to prioritize whole, naturally gluten-free foods, and treat processed options as occasional additions to your diet rather than staples.

How do I handle travel with celiac disease?

When traveling with celiac disease, planning is crucial for maintaining a gluten-free diet. Before your trip, research gluten-free dining options and grocery stores at your destination. Pack gluten-free snacks to have on hand in case suitable food is not available during your travels.

Communicate your dietary restrictions to airline staff or hotel personnel, and consider carrying a gluten-free travel card in the local language to make dining out easier. Being proactive in your planning helps ensure you can enjoy your trip without the stress of potential gluten exposure.

Can I eat out safely?

Eating out with celiac disease requires careful planning and communication with restaurant staff. Always choose restaurants that are familiar with gluten-free dining practices. Before visiting, check the menu online to identify gluten-free options, and call ahead to discuss your dietary needs with the restaurant.

When dining, clearly communicate your gluten intolerance to your server and inquire about food preparation methods to avoid cross-contamination. Request that your meal be prepared in a separate area using clean utensils. This proactive approach helps ensure a safer dining experience while enjoying meals away from home.

How do I educate my family and friends?

Educating family and friends about celiac disease is essential for creating a supportive environment. Start by explaining what celiac disease is, how it affects your health, and the importance of avoiding gluten. Provide them with resources, such as brochures or reputable websites, that offer additional information about the condition.

Encourage open dialogue about your dietary needs during gatherings or meals. Sharing recipes and gluten-free cooking tips can help them understand how to accommodate your needs while also enjoying meals together. Making them partners in your journey fosters understanding and reduces the likelihood of accidental gluten exposure.

Detailed FAQs

1. What is the difference between celiac disease and gluten sensitivity?

Celiac disease is an autoimmune condition where the ingestion of gluten leads to damage in the small intestine. This damage can result in a variety of symptoms, including gastrointestinal distress, fatigue, and nutrient deficiencies. On the other hand, gluten sensitivity does not involve an autoimmune response or intestinal damage; it can cause symptoms similar to those of celiac disease but without the same health risks.

To differentiate between the two, it's essential to seek professional medical advice. A healthcare provider can conduct tests to determine if your symptoms stem from celiac disease or gluten sensitivity. Understanding this distinction is crucial for managing your diet and health effectively.

2. How is celiac disease diagnosed?

Celiac disease is primarily diagnosed through a series of blood tests that check for specific antibodies associated with the condition. If these tests indicate a likelihood of celiac disease, your doctor may recommend an intestinal biopsy to assess damage to the villi, the tiny hair-like structures in the small intestine that absorb nutrients.

It's vital to remain on a gluten-containing diet until you've completed these tests to ensure accurate results. After diagnosis, your healthcare provider will guide you on the next steps, which typically include adopting a strict gluten-free diet to manage the condition.

3. What should I do if I think I have celiac disease?

If you suspect you have celiac disease, the first step is to consult a healthcare provider. They will conduct the necessary tests to confirm the diagnosis before you make any significant dietary changes. Avoiding gluten prematurely can affect test results, so it's essential to seek medical advice first.

Once diagnosed, your healthcare provider will help you understand how to transition to a gluten-free diet. They may refer you to a dietitian who specializes in celiac disease for tailored dietary advice, ensuring you meet your nutritional needs while avoiding gluten.

4. Are all gluten-free foods safe?

Not all gluten-free foods are automatically safe for those with celiac disease. While they may not contain gluten, cross-contamination during production or preparation can pose a risk. Always look for products labeled with a certified gluten-free seal to ensure they meet safety standards.

Additionally, read ingredient lists carefully, as some products may contain hidden gluten. It's also wise to ask about food preparation methods when dining out to avoid potential cross-contamination. Being vigilant about food safety is crucial in managing your health.

5. Can I eat oats?

You can include oats in your gluten-free diet, but only if they are certified gluten-free. Oats are often grown and processed in facilities that also handle gluten-containing grains, leading to a high risk of cross-contamination. Look for brands that specifically state they are gluten-free.

When starting to incorporate oats, do so gradually and monitor your body's response. If you experience any symptoms, consult your healthcare provider to determine if oats are suitable for your individual dietary needs. Always prioritize certified gluten-free options to ensure safety.